The Keto Diet Damaged Our Health

A Better Approach

David Klein

ISBN-13: 978-1729613511
ISBN-10: 1729613519

Edited by David Klein
Cover Design by PixelStudios and David Klein
Cover Photo: Marian Weyo/Shutterstock.com
Mediterranean Pyramid Image: Oldways, www.oldwayspt.org

DISCLAIMER: This book is intended as an educational tool only and is not intended to provide personal medical advice. Rather, it's a book that teaches the principles of sound nutrition. If you have a medical issue or are looking for medical advice, or if you believe that you need to make dietary changes to improve your health, it is recommended that you consult with a qualified physician.

david@davidkleinwriting.com
www.davidkleinwriting.com

Acknowledgement

This book is dedicated to my favorite person on this entire planet, my wife and best friend Rae. Not only does Rae Rae not know that I'm writing this dedication, she doesn't even know that I'm writing or publishing this book. I'm going to surprise her with the book and dedication as part of a gift for our upcoming 35th wedding anniversary. (Note to florist: If she doesn't like the book, please get something ready, and fast.)

I can't even begin to describe how proud I am of Rae. Her priorities are just right, she's kind and sweet, and everyone seems to love her. I love what I teasingly call Rae's "cackle sessions": she talks to her friends on the phone and they laugh and laugh, usually with that laughter escalating in volume and frequency as the conversation goes on. I can't hear what she's saying, but it doesn't matter; that happy sound fills my heart with joy. She's also just about the epitome of industriousness. Part of that is her work as an editor. But she's not touching this book until it's published. She deserves to get a book from me, at least once, in finished form. And as I've said in every book I've ever published, Rae is the funniest person I've ever known. She's made me laugh so hard that I've had to pull off the highway because I couldn't see the road anymore. (Note to Misty, our State Farm agent: You didn't read that.)

And just one quick story, going back almost 35 years. Rae is very athletic, and I'd like to tell you about the greatest catch she ever made . . . me. Please stop rolling your eyes, because that's not what I meant . . . When we were newly married, I was up on a roof cleaning a window. The roof's surface had gotten wet with the slippery cleaning solution, and I started to slide down. Gravity had taken over and there was no turning back. Rae saw it happen and like a trained baseball fielder she yelled: "I've got you." Sure enough, she caught me before I hit the ground. I'll never know, but I might be limping to this day if she hadn't done that. (Note to clumsy people: Stay off roofs.)

Thank you, Rae Rae, for everything. Words alone can't capture your excellence and beauty as a wife and friend. Not only do I love you, but I really, really, like you. (Note to self: Never, ever, let her forget that I feel this way. She deserves to hear it every day.)

Table of Contents

Introduction

Some time ago, my endocrinologist suggested that I consider trying the newly popular ketogenic diet. He said to do "deep research" to see if I thought the diet might work for me. And that's what I did. I was amazed to find such a wealth of information on the web and in published books about the newly popular "keto diet," as it's commonly referred to.

Why did my doctor suggest keto for me? I was somewhat overweight, but the main reason was that I was having energy problems. For forty years I've suffered with severe adrenal fatigue syndrome, where I've had to eat frequently to keep my strength up. Often a half-hour after eating I was hungry again and feeling drained and light-headed. My doctor explained that I might not be efficient at processing carbohydrates, and that the keto diet changes the body from a carbohydrate burning machine to a fat burning machine.

After a few days of research I was sold. I immediately began easing into the keto diet, which represented a dramatic change from my previous diet. (Some jump right into the keto diet full force, but that usually comes with what is called the "keto flu," which mirrors many symptoms of the literal flu. Voluntary flu? No thank you.) I made the change over about a three-week period.

What happened? The transition phase was slightly uncomfortable, but at the same time it was rewarding and exciting. And very soon I was enjoying the diet immensely. My wife, who decided to join me on keto, began making lots of delicious high-fat foods. We were enjoying scones with icing, deliciously sweetened with carbohydrate-free Swerve, and many other similar goodies, including lots of items made with heavy cream. And while we ate to satisfaction, the pounds started to melt off. I lost 14 pounds in six weeks, and I wasn't really trying to lose weight. My wife also lost a little weight, though she really didn't need to. (See,

I'm establishing myself as no dummy right out of the blocks.) We both became enthralled with our new foods, a feeling of calm, and we even somehow enjoyed testing for ketones, which involved finger-sticks to test blood. It was an exciting time with lots of high expectations. We knew we were ketoers for life.

But in about two months we both decided to stop the keto diet, and for similar reasons. Here's why:

After my wife, Rae, began the keto diet, she began to feel increasingly sluggish. She simply didn't feel good and had less energy and vitality than she did before going keto. She said that her skin and muscle tone lacked vitality. Even her fingernails seemed to be affected, as she noticed a ridging pattern that was not there before. She found that she was going to the gym less frequently and staying for shorter amounts of time, because she needed to conserve what little energy she had. I encouraged her to be patient, to stick with it, and to increase her carbs a little bit. The more she increased her carb intake, the better she felt. Finally, when she had increased her carbs to above what is allowed on the keto diet, she began to feel like she wanted to: energized and ready to meet each day's demands. She stopped the keto diet completely, and during the next few months she reported a progressive improvement: she felt better and better, and her energy levels returned to normal. Her skin, muscle tone, and fingernails returned to their pre-keto condition. She is very happy to be off the keto diet and back on a healthy, balanced diet.

My story is similar. Once I transitioned to the keto diet, I was in it full force: I read about the keto diet every day, and I adhered to the diet closely. I kept my carb levels as low as possible, which was probably between 25 and 50 grams of net carbs a day. I felt good in a way, and not so good in a way. The Good: Keeping my carb levels low, essentially breaking a carbohydrate addiction, brought a feeling of peace. No more wild swings in blood sugar levels, with the resulting highs and lows of energy spurts and the soon to follow energy drains. The Bad: While my energy was steadier, it was now at a lower level overall. I found myself going to the gym much less often, and when I did go I spent less time there and expended less energy. (My time with resistance training decreased, and my time in the massage chair increased.) I stayed home more, I worked less, and I frequently opted not to go out of the home to care for necessary tasks.

The Worst: I have a long history of severe adrenal fatigue syndrome, with adrenal crashes, which are periods of extreme low energy where the body essentially enters survival mode and all systems are on partial shutdown. The body enters this state because the adrenal glands, which secrete several known hormones that help to supply and regulate energy, are now unable to supply the necessary fuels that power the body.

Severe adrenal crashes are kind of like the flu without the fever. The body becomes so weak that even the smallest task, such as standing up, seems daunting and exhausting. For some, complete bed rest is needed for a couple of days to begin the recovery process. And yes, I've been there many times.

Cortisol is probably the most important of the adrenal hormones. Cortisol is referred to as the "stress hormone," and when your adrenal glands become exhausted and can no longer match your body's needs for cortisol . . . here comes the crash. I've been taking prescription hydrocortisone for about six years, on what is called a "replacement dose". This is not a case of trying to steroid up, but rather to supply the amount of cortisol that the body would normally make if the adrenal glands were healthy. And this therapy had basically stopped my crashes. I hadn't had a severe adrenal crash for about five years.

After about six weeks on the keto diet, the crashes returned, and they were severe. The littlest stress would bring on a crash. I had about four crashes in a two-week period, and then I realized that the keto diet was causing them. I was literally starving my body of the fuel it needed to avoid and overcome the crash, and no amount of cortisone would stop those crashes. So two months into keto I stopped the diet, and the adrenal crashes immediately lessened.

At that time I began an intensive study of health, nutrition, and diet. Part of that was to look at the keto diet from the other angle—that of why it is not a healthy and balanced diet. The research I found was quite striking. But I also spent much time reviewing the healthiest diets in the world, thus renewing and reviving an interest that I've had my entire life: how to live in the most healthful manner possible.

In this book I share with you the results of that research. And I discuss the positives and negatives of the keto diet, as well as offer a better, healthier, more logical, reasonable, natural, and balanced approach to diet and sound health.

David Klein
November, 2018

What is the Keto Diet?

The ketogenic diet, most often known as the "keto diet" or simply as "keto", is, in a way, relatively new. It actually came into existence in the 1920s as a treatment for epilepsy. But in the last couple of years, beginning about 2016, it's gained great popularity among the general population as a weight-loss diet. It seems to be exploding in popularity as I write this in the year 2018. There's now an abundance of how-to keto books and recipe books on the market. We're talking hundreds of them, if not thousands. (And if there are not yet literally thousands of keto books, give it a year or two more, and there probably will be. It seems that one is being published almost daily.)

There are slight variations in the keto diet, depending upon the author's interpretation of the diet, but all variations have this in common: The keto diet is one that is very low in carbohydrates, moderate in protein, and very high in fat. Protein intake is not given much attention, but the two key components of keto are that the diet must be very low in carbohydrates and very high in fat.

But wait, doesn't eating fat make the body fat? Keto experts are quick to point out that eating fat does not make the body fat; it's eating too many carbohydrates, especially in the forms of sugars and starches, that cause the body to make and store excessive fat cells. Are those experts correct? Yes, they are. Eating excessive carbohydrates, and especially sugars and starches, will likely pack on the pounds, and quickly.

Here's A Synopsis of How the Keto Diet Works:

The human body is designed to run on, or burn, two main types of fuels: sugar and fat. All forms of carbohydrates break down to sugar (glucose) before they are used as fuel. What is the body's first choice of fuel when both sugar and fat are available? Typically sugar. It's easier to burn and the body will keep burning sugar first as long as it's available, especially during moderate to strenuous activity. Sugar is quick fuel, and it gets priority status.

But when sugar is not available, the body is forced to burn fat. And that's the key component in the keto diet: Severely restrict carbs, cutting off the sugar supply, and the body has no choice but to burn fat.

As I mentioned, there are many variations in the keto diet. Most of the variation is in the amount of carbohydrates that are allowed. Typically, most keto diets allow up to 50 grams of net carbohydrates a day. Some restrict the total to 20-30 grams of net carbohydrates a day. The most severe I've ever seen, and I really mean severe, is an allowance of a maximum of 20 grams of TOTAL carbohydrates a day.

You may be wondering what the difference is between NET carbohydrates and TOTAL carbohydrates. Total carbohydrates refer to all forms of carbohydrates: There are different types of carbohydrates, such as simple and complex. Simple carbohydrates refer to sugars, whereas complex carbohydrates refer to carbohydrates other than sugar that need to be broken down by the body into sugar (glucose) before they can be used as fuel. Then there are fibers, which are also counted as carbohydrates. Fibers, however, are not digestible by the body, so they don't raise the blood sugar level. Finally, there are sugar alcohols. These add sweetness to food, but they act in the body as neither sugar nor alcohol. They do not burn as fuels and they do not add to the blood sugar or alcohol levels. Sugar alcohols are commonly found in low-carb protein bars and drinks. Common sugar alcohols are sorbitol, mannitol, xylitol, maltitol, lactitol, and erythritol.

So what are net carbs? They are the total carbs minus the fiber and sugar alcohols. Since neither fiber nor sugar alcohol increases the blood sugar level, neither is counted as a net carb. So when you read labels, make sure to do the math and subtract any fiber (soluble or insoluble) and sugar alcohols from the total amount of carbs. This will yield the net carb total.

Why is it called the "ketogenic" or "keto" diet?

We've learned that when carbohydrates are severely restricted, the body has no choice but to begin burning fats. These fats are burned from two sources: the fats in the foods we eat and also the fat cells stored in the body. When fats are burned, a substance called "ketones" is produced and sent to the bloodstream: it's actually the ketones that are supplying the body's fuel.

So the name keto is a descriptive name for the diet. Restrict carbohydrates and fat is burned, which makes ketones. Those ketones are burned as energy by the body. When the ketone count reaches a certain level, the body is said to be in "ketosis."

But wait, I've heard that being in ketosis is dangerous. Is it?

What you've probably heard is that a related condition that can afflict diabetics, called "ketoacidosis", is dangerous. Ketoacidosis occurs when the ketone levels become extremely high. Actually, the word "dangerous" is an understatement: severe ketoacidosis can be deadly to diabetics. But most people are in no danger of going into a state of ketoacidosis. It's the conditions of diabetes that bring on ketoacidosis. (Others who may be in danger of going into ketoacidosis are those who are severely ill, alcoholics, and those who are literally starving.)

The goal of the keto diet is for the dieter to have ketone levels consistently in the range of 0.5 to 3.0 mmol/L. While those levels mean that the body is, to a degree, in minor starvation mode (and that's why it's burning a lot of fat), actually ketoacidosis does not begin until the levels exceed what is considered safe for the keto diet. When levels are greater than 3.0 mmol/L, it's usually prudent to seek medical attention.

For the average person on the keto diet, reaching such high levels of ketones is not usually a problem. For the two months I was on the diet, my highest ketone reading was, I believe, 1.2 mmol/L. My average was perhaps 0.6 mmol/L.

Before beginning any diet, it's usually the course of wisdom to check with your physician, who may know something about your condition that makes a particular diet an unwise choice for you.

Does that mean that the keto diet is a good choice?

Probably not. An upcoming chapter will answer the question: What's Wrong with the Keto Diet?

I've heard it said that the keto diet is a "starvation diet". Is that true?

Not really, but it is, to a degree, partially true. A starvation diet, by definition, is eating nothing at all for a prolonged period of time. But it can also refer to a diet that severely restricts caloric intake for a prolonged period of time.

Those on the keto diet are allowed to eat many rich and fatty foods, and they can eat them to satisfaction as often as they like. Caloric intake can actually be quite high, and being on the diet can even be fun. (High-fat foods with today's artificial sweeteners can taste surprisingly like the real thing.) So no, the keto diet is not a starvation diet.

However, one of the three macronutrients, carbohydrates, is severely restricted on the keto diet. So while the body has an abundance of fats and enough proteins, it is, to a degree, starving for carbohydrates. It's this process that makes your body burn fat and thus lose weight.

Summary of the Keto Diet

The keto diet is very high in fat and very low in carbohydrates. By being low in carbohydrates, the body is forced to burn fat as fuel. When fat is burned, it produces ketones, and it is the ketones that are actually used as fuel by the body. Hence, the name keto diet.

Does the Keto Diet Work?

Yes, the keto diet works very well. No, the keto diet does not work. Which is the correct answer, yes or no? Actually, both are correct . . . it just depends on what you are looking for in a diet. Is your goal weight loss or is it vibrant health (which often includes weight loss)?

The main claim of keto proponents is that being on the keto diet will cause you to lose weight. Does it do that? Yes, very well. By restricting carbohydrate intake, the body is forced to burn fat cells. Most people who adhere to the keto diet will lose weight, and they will do so quickly.

Note: Weight loss will be especially rapid during the first ten days or so on the keto diet. That is because when you severely restrict carbohydrate intake, your muscles will lose most of their store of glycogen. (When you eat carbohydrates, the fuel that is not used immediately is converted to glycogen, which is stored in the muscles and liver for later use as energy.) Glycogen carries water. So as your glycogen stores diminish, your weight goes down. It's not uncommon to lose six or more pounds in the first two weeks on the keto diet. But please keep in mind that during this phase, most of your weight loss will be water weight, along with a little fat and perhaps even a little muscle. (So if you lose six pounds in the first two weeks, probably about four of those pounds are water weight, and the other two pounds are mostly fat stores.)

If you remain on the keto diet, and you are faithful to it, you may lose an additional one to two pounds per week. You can do this while actually eating a normal amount of food. Again, the keto diet puts the body in fat-burning mode, or survival mode, if you will, and fat can just melt off.

That sounds great, doesn't it? So why did I also write that the keto diet doesn't work? It's important to note that weight loss and vibrant health are not necessarily synonymous. Just because you are losing weight does not mean that you are improving your overall health. While maintaining proper weight is an important factor in obtaining good health, it is not the ONLY factor. And this is where the keto diet usually falls short. I'll discuss the shortcomings of the keto diet in an upcoming chapter.

What Else is Appealing about the Keto Diet?

1. People love fad diets.

It's no secret that people tend to flock, en mass, to fad diets. Many of these diets are popular for a time, often with millions adhering to them, and their founders gaining fame and wealth. People on these diets have both their successes and their failures, and then a new diet becomes the new fad . . . until the next fad diet hits the scene. And the keto diet will likely prove to be like the rest of the fad diets. (I'm so aware of this trend that I feel pressure to complete and publish this book while the keto diet is still the fad diet. I'm fully aware that in a year or two the keto diet may go the way of the Atkins Diet, the Ornish Diet, and the Pritikin Diet.)

Anyone buy a Pritikin diet book recently? While the Pritikin Diet was the rage in the early 1980s, if you were not living and an adult at that time, have you even ever heard of Nathan Pritikin or his Pritikin Diet? Obviously my spell-checker hasn't, because it just flagged the spelling of "Pritikin" as unknown. Interestingly, it did not flag the word "keto." But in 1980, when the Pritikin Diet was in its heyday, it would have surely recognized the spelling "Pritikin" and flagged the term "keto" as unknown . . . To quote a line from one of my favorite movies: "Out with the old and in with the new."

2. Rapid initial weight loss.

The keto diet, and any other low-carb diet, gets a huge boost from the fact that weight loss takes place so rapidly. As I mentioned in a previous chapter, weight loss comes very rapidly on these diets, because as carbohydrate intake is reduced, glycogen stores in the muscles and liver quickly diminish, and glycogen carries water. So even though most of the initial weight loss from the keto diet is water weight, there's no denying the excitement generated as the numbers on the scale go down. We are driven by success, and quick weight loss on the keto diet is very motivating.

3. A couple of good philosophies.

The keto diet preaches several philosophies that are true, and you won't hear these philosophies much outside of the keto diet. One is that "dietary fats are not the enemy." It's kind of a shame that dietary fat and body fat have the same name: "fat," because it's easy to make the implication that eating fat makes the body fat. That simply is not true. In fact, for most people, if they ate a diet exclusively of fat they would begin to lose weight rapidly. (And they'd get seriously ill just as rapidly.) It's eating excessive carbohydrates that causes the body to store fat. Fats are an important part of a healthy diet, and they are not the enemy.

Another philosophy of keto proponents is a message to those who are overweight: "It's not your fault." For the most part, this is true. There has been such a confusing and conflicting cyclone of dietary information released and preached in our lifetimes that even a brilliant person would be overwhelmed.

I've been such a victim myself. For many years I adhered to low-fat diets, thinking that these would bring increased vitality and health. As I look back I see a correlation between these diets and my waistline. The moment I began to eat a low-fat diet is the moment that I began to gain belly weight. I'm not alone in this dilemma: the same thing has happened to countless millions of others. In my case, in just a few years I went from being trim to overweight to the point that a young friend of mine, C.C., would put her hand on my stomach and say things like: "I think I feel the baby kicking." Cute C.C.!

Note: Why do low-fat diets tend to make a person gain body fat?

Is it the low fat content itself that makes a person fat? No. Here's what happens: When a person goes on a low-fat diet, they need to replace the previous dietary calories with something else, and there are only three caloric choices left: Protein, Carbohydrates, and Alcohol. Increasing alcohol consumption is not, of course, a good idea. Most people will increase both protein and carbohydrates, and usually carbs get preference. It's the increase in carbohydrates that causes one to begin to pack on body fat. The increase in carbohydrates causes the blood sugar to rise, which prompts the body to make an excessive amount of insulin. Insulin has been called "the fat storing hormone." As insulin levels rise in the bloodstream, more fat will be stored in the body.

4. Quick testing results.

Ketone production can appear on home testing systems just a day or two after beginning the diet. Further, you can be "in ketosis," which is your goal, just as quickly. That alone can be very motivating. There are three methods of testing for ketones: 1. Urine strips. 2. A breathalyzer. 3. Blood tests, via finger stick, which is very similar to the method used for testing blood glucose levels. Are all three methods equally effective? No. Urine strips are unreliable, a breathalyzer is somewhat accurate, and blood tests are very accurate. When the blood ketone levels reach 0.5 mmol/L, you are said to be in ketosis. Levels of ketones between 0.5 and 3.0 mmol/L are considered safe—the higher the level, the more fat you are burning and the more ketones you are producing.

Again, testing for ketones can be very gratifying. Think about a person who is trying to lose weight, and their goal is perhaps to lose, say, forty pounds. When the scale shows they've lost three pounds, it's a feeling of slight accomplishment, but it's also very frustrating to see how far they still have to go . . . many months if not a year or years. But with ketone readings, if your goal is to be in ketosis at 0.5 mmol/L or greater, you can reach that goal in a day or two. Reaching that goal is very satisfying.

So is the Keto Diet a Healthy, Balanced Diet?

Simply put, no, it's not. *The U.S. News and World Report* conducted a comprehensive study and comparison of 40 of the most popular diets in 2018. Under the category of Best Diet for Healthy Eating, where did the panel of experts rank the keto diet? Dead last, at number 40.

The keto diet is a gimmick diet, like so many others before it. What makes it a gimmick diet? It takes shortcuts to achieve a goal, but it is not in harmony with known and respected sound nutritional principles—in fact, it flies in the face of those principles. It's a focusing on a tree of good health and not the entire forest.

What's Wrong with the Keto Diet?

Plenty. While the keto diet will likely help you to lose weight, it will not benefit your overall health, and it may even damage your health. There are other ways to lose weight that will boost your vitality and that have no known shortcomings.

The keto diet is based on partial knowledge, and partial knowledge can be misleading. For instance, here is a true statement: When I was in high school, I played on the football team, and to this day I still hold the national record (U.S.) for highest percentage of passes completed in a high school career. Well, actually, I'm tied for the record.

Again, that is a true statement. Based on that one fact, you may be viewing me as a star quarterback with a stellar arm. In reality, mine was a chicken arm if there ever was one, and I didn't even play quarterback. I played end, and I threw only one pass in high school, a slow, high-arching wobble ball, that happened to be during a trick play to a wide open receiver. So yes, technically I'm tied for the record of completions at 100 percent with my one pass, but the thought of me as an outstanding quarterback is laughable. (And indeed, my head coach did laugh at me after the game about that feeble-looking throw.) I was anything but a quarterback. That one statistic was misleading because it didn't paint the entire picture.

And thus is the case with the keto diet. The weight loss is undeniable, and is a positive, but that's not the complete picture. There are too many negatives to the diet, things that detract from overall well-being, that make the diet unhealthful. Let's look at a few of them.

1. The keto diet is hyper-focused on macronutrients: micronutrients are all but ignored.

What are macronutrients and what are micronutrients? There are three macronutrients: proteins, carbohydrates, and fats. The keto diet's main feature is the balance of the three macronutrients: fats comprise a high percentage of the diet, proteins comprise a moderate percentage of the diet, and carbohydrates are severely restricted and kept at a minimum.

But micronutrients are just as important as macronutrients: micronutrients refer to vitamins and minerals. Enzymes and other factors in food are also important. Dietitians have known for years that abundant and varied micronutrients are a key to good health. For instance, *Harvard Health Publishing*, Harvard Medical School, September 2016, reported: "To maintain your brain, muscle, bone, nerves, skin, blood circulation, and immune system, your body requires a steady supply of many different raw materials—both macronutrients and micronutrients. You need large amounts of macronutrients—proteins, fats, and carbohydrates. And while you only need a small number of micronutrients—vitamins and minerals—failing to get even those small quantities virtually guarantees disease." But again, the keto diet minimizes the importance of micronutrients. The focus is clearly on macronutrients.

As an example, carrots are a known powerhouse of micronutrients. Especially are they high in healthful fibers, beta carotene, and other vitamins and minerals. But on the keto diet, carrots are either severely restricted or even listed as "to be avoided." At the same time, bacon, which has never enjoyed the best reputation in health circles, to say the least, is a glorified food on the keto diet. On keto, you can eat as much bacon as you want. Some keto dieters actually where t-shirts glorifying bacon. In what rational world is bacon a health food and carrots are not?

2. The keto diet is loaded with a big no-no: empty calories.

Foods such as butter, heavy cream, bacon, sour cream, mayonnaise, and others are highly encouraged on the keto diet. But while these foods supply an abundance of fat and calories, they are lacking in nutrients. A healthful diet should be nutrient rich, or nutrient dense, and those foods are not. We are probably all familiar with the term "bang for your buck." The keto diet is loaded with foods that provide little nutritional bang.

3. Keto proponents claim that you can burn EITHER sugars or fats, one at a time, but not both. That's simply not true.

The human body is amazing. The details of its functions, from large to microscopic, are astounding. And the body's "wisdom" is marvelous. It knows when to burn sugars and when to burn fats. To make sure it does that, we just need to learn to live in accordance with its functions and rhythms, supplying it with the proper nutrients, exercise, and rest.

The keto diet is more or less a trick on the body. Starve the body of carbohydrates and it will be forced to burn fat. But the fact is, you don't need to starve the body of carbohydrates to burn fat. If you eat the proper amount of carbohydrates, your body can use what it needs when it needs it. Especially each night, when you are asleep and abstaining from food for 7-10 hours, the body will burn enough fat to keep your weight at normal levels. That's really the ideal eating plan. Eat enough carbs to enjoy vibrant health . . . but not so many that you store extra fat.

Your body doesn't come with an external on-off switch for burning sugars and fats; that wisdom is built in. If you eat wisely, the body knows when to burn sugar and when to burn fat.

4. Keto proponents are quick to point out that the keto diet should be avoided by two groups: children and serious athletes.

That may be a true statement, but . . . I find that truth, that serious athletes and children should not be on the keto diet, rather, well, laughable. Why? Because I don't know about you, but I want to be on the diet that children and athletes are on. Whatever it is that's fueling them with such great energy, I want that too. The keto diet, by severely limiting carbohydrate consumption, is seriously under fueled.

5. Overall, the keto diet does not adhere to the principles of good nutrition.

Through the years, nutritionists have identified many tried-and-true principles of sound nutrition. The keto diet all but ignores some of these principles, and it goes directly against others. Let's look at a few of these principles.

a. Fruit. Fruit clearly has a special place in the human diet. There's a wonderful variety of colors and flavors, and fruit is very energizing, cleansing, and is filled with vitamins, minerals, enzymes, fibers, and other healthful substances. It's estimated that there are 2,000 different types of fruits on this planet. And there are way, way more varieties. For instance, there are now 7,500 varieties of apples. Apples are clearly a wonderful dietary gift. On the keto diet, you can eat maybe one apple per day and then no other fruit. (Some varieties of apples will, just by eating one, push you over the carbohydrate limit for the entire day on the keto diet.) Let's say you love apples and decide to try each of the 7,500 varieties. At one apple per day, that would take you over twenty years on the keto diet. And if you like bananas just as much and want to do the same with those, that's another four years. Do the words "unreasonable restriction" begin to come to mind here?

I mentioned earlier that my wife Rae and I spent two months on the keto diet. Berries are just about the only fruit that is allowed without severe restriction. We did our keto diet in May and June, and berries were abundant. One of us made the comment to the other: 'What are we going to do when berries go out of season soon?' It was like we had to wait the entire year to eat fresh fruits again. That's just plain silly.

Fruits are a major part of the summer harvest. From a dietary point of view, it's a special time here on Earth. With the keto carbohydrate severe restriction, fruits are not allowed to take their natural place in our diets.

b. Fiber. In recent decades the marvelous role of fiber has been identified and appreciated by nutritionists. Fiber is necessary for the health of our digestive system. Soluble fiber absorbs liquid and adds helpful bulk to stools. Insoluble fiber helps to push things through the digestive system. Thus, when you eat enough fiber, digestion is much more efficient, which means that you'll feel better, have more energy, and will be at a lower risk for cancers of the digestive system, including colon cancer. Fiber also regulates blood sugar and lowers cholesterol.

The keto diet is so focused on fats and so minimizes carbohydrates that most of the foods that provide fibers are either restricted or prohibited. We are talking about healthful foods like beans, grains, and fruits.

c. High fat. Diets that are high in dietary fat, especially when those fat sources are animal-based, have long been considered dangerous. High-fat diets are especially harmful to cardiovascular health. The keto diet is loaded with fats, and most of those fats tend to come from animal sources, which are high in saturated fat.

6. Your adrenal glands will become strained and eventually exhausted.

If your adrenal glands become exhausted, that means that YOU have become exhausted. Your adrenal glands supply lots of spark to your system by secreting cortisol and adrenaline, as well as other substances. You can think of your adrenal glands as your body's battery.

So how does the keto diet strain and exhaust your adrenal glands? The answer is actually quite simple. Your body needs lots of fuel to handle each day's demands. Your fuel comes from three primary sources: your food intake, your energy stores of glycogen in both the muscles and liver, and stored fat. When you eat, some of your food is used as immediate energy and the rest is stored as either glycogen in the muscles and liver or as body fat. Primarily, the fuels from food and glycogen are energizing your body. When food and stored glycogen are not available, your body will begin to burn fat, which you'll recall is the premise of the keto diet in the first place. But fat energy is not quick energy, it burns slowly and is utilized slowly. That works great at night when you are asleep, but when you are working and playing, your body needs lots of quick fuel. Where does it get that quick fuel if sugar and glycogen are not readily available? Enter the adrenal glands, which will respond by pumping out copious amounts of energy in the form of adrenal hormones, most notably cortisol and adrenaline.

The adrenal glands were meant to work in a backup role, supplying energy as needed in short bursts. But on the keto diet, the adrenal glands take on a full-time role. They must work hard all day long to supply the missing energy from a lack of carbohydrates and glycogen. Like any gland, organ, or muscle that is overstressed for a period of time, exhaustion is inevitable.

You'll recall that even the most lenient versions of the keto diet max out at fifty grams of carbohydrates per day. While each person has different needs, most need at least 75 to 90 grams per day to supply the body the minimal amount of fuel it needs to function. So the keto diet, with its carbohydrate limit, overworks the adrenal glands and almost guarantees their eventual exhaustion. When this happens, I promise, you will not be happy. And the road to recovery can be long, painful, expensive, and very frustrating.

7. You'll gain the water weight back as soon as you leave the keto diet.

That fabulously quick weight loss that was so encouraging at the start of the keto diet is likely mostly temporary. Most of the pounds that are shed at the start of the keto diet, or any severely restricted carbohydrate diet, are simply water weight. That happens because your glycogen stores in the muscles and liver are used up and not replenished, and glycogen carries water. If you leave the keto diet, all that glycogen, with its water weight, will come back just as quickly as it left.

8. The keto diet can cause serious health issues.

Interestingly, most of the authors who write keto diet and cookbooks are NOT health professionals. They are average people who tried the diet, lost weight, and got so "into keto" that they began to tell all their friends about the diet, collect recipes, and ultimately write books. But medical professionals have compiled a long list of potential health problems from any high-fat, low-carb diet. Here's a list of some of those issues:

Heart Disease
Hypertension
Constipation
Diarrhea
Loss of Lean Muscle Mass

Poor Complexion
Vitamin Deficiency
Decreased Metabolism
Low Blood Sugar
Nutritional Deficiencies
Loss of Electrolytes
Dehydration
Light Headedness
Kidney Stones
Kidney Damage
Bad Breath
Liver Problems
Dizziness
Weight Regain (when leaving the diet)
Lack of Energy
Lack of Motivation
Fertility Issues
Adrenal Gland Stress and Fatigue

Keep in mind that the popularity of the keto diet is recent, keto having become the "in diet" just the last few years. Oftentimes, it takes several months or years adhering to a diet before deficiencies and medical problems surface. According to Hilary Brueck, diet expert and science reporter for *Business Insider*: "Banning entire food groups and thinking you can cheat your way into good health may work for a while, but it could also send you into an early grave." Time will tell how many problems arise from the keto diet and the level of their severity. Then again, my wife and I, as well as many others, can attest to the fact that some of the above problems can be experienced in a very short time on the keto diet.

Clearly, the keto diet has one main benefit: weight loss. But there are other ways to lose weight that don't compromise your health. Weight loss is like a single tree in the forest of good health. Don't ignore those other trees; they are important too. Some of those trees may be bearing apples, peaches, oranges, and the like. The fruitage of those trees are literally beautiful, healthful, and delicious. It would be foolish for most people to shun them.

In summary, the keto diet, in many ways, completely ignores the time-tested principles of good nutrition. For instance, there is a mountain of evidence from highly respected sources and studies that show that excessive saturated fats are damaging to the cardiovascular system. Yet, the keto diet is loaded with saturated fats.

Keto proponents act like this vast amount of research never existed in the first place. It reminds me of something we've seen from time to time with aged ex-professional athletes. The scenario is this: A player who was a star in his prime, and then watched his skills deteriorate with age until he could no longer compete and had to retire, announces perhaps five or even ten years later that he is making a comeback. Those "comebacks" always end in a sad manner. The athlete finds that his skills have further deteriorated and he is completely overmatched. He forgot that the very reason he had to leave the game was that his skills deteriorated with age. Did he think that the laws of aging no longer applied to him? Did he think that when he made his comeback he would be younger than when he retired?

And such is the keto diet. Proponents can choose to ignore the long established principles of good nutrition, but that doesn't mean that they won't eventually reap the results of their decision. Just as aged athletes can't ignore away the effects of time on the human body, keto dieters can't ignore away the mountain of research of sound nutritional principles. (They can ignore it, but they can't ignore it <u>away</u>.)

A Better Approach to Diet

Is there a better approach to diet than keto? Absolutely. I'll list the principles and suggestions, and then I'll describe a few of the best diets for your health:

1. The human body is very wise. Don't try to fool it, such as with a fad diet, but work in harmony with it.

Experts in the field of nutrition have given much advice as to what constitutes a healthy diet. Some of those "experts" are way out there in left field, and others know what they are talking about. Among those who know what they're talking about, there is one common thread, and this thread has endured decades of fad diets and other crazy eating notions. What is that thread? Our diets should be based on foods that are healthy, unprocessed, and in their natural state as much as possible. Eat a wide variety of healthful foods for better health.

2. Eat a balance of proteins, fats, and carbohydrates. (The three macronutrients)

Regarding proteins, fats, and carbohydrates, there are no bad guys. They are the three essential macronutrients, and they all play vital roles in building vibrant health. You need all three not only to function well, but to live. As long as the macronutrients are kept in reasonable balance and eaten in healthful forms, you can achieve better health.

So what is a proper balance of the three macronutrients? Of course, that can vary in individuals to some degree. However, since the principles of nutrition are sound and universal, the variance should not be a wild swing.

Some diet experts recommend that you achieve balanced meals in a way that is simpler and often more practical than counting grams of the various macronutrients. Here's how: You visually fill your plate with the proper proportions. They suggest filling half of your plate with non-starchy vegetables, such as salad, broccoli, asparagus, sautéed spinach, and so on; one-quarter of your plate with protein, such as fish, meat, or eggs; and one-quarter of your plate with healthy carbohydrates, such as a starchy vegetable, grain, or beans. What about fats? You should include some fats with each meal, which slow down the absorption of carbohydrates and leave you feeling satisfied for a longer time after the meal. Some proteins will supply fats, such as salmon or grass-fed beef. If your protein portion does not supply fat, you can also add some olive oil or some nuts or seeds to boost fat content.

3. "Eat the Rainbow." (The micronutrients)

Eat the rainbow? That's an odd saying. What does it mean? As we look in nature, we see there is an abundance of healthful, natural foods that grow out of the ground. And those foods come in all colors and many shades of those colors. Hence, the term "eat the rainbow" refers to eating a wide variety of natural foods. By doing this, you will likely be eating foods of all the colors in the rainbow. This is the foundation of a healthful diet, as it practically assures that you'll be getting the greatest amount of healthy micronutrients from your food that you realistically can.

A sample rainbow of foods (the rainbow's colors are red, orange, yellow, green, blue, indigo, and violet):

Red: Cherries, Cranberries, Kidney Beans, Tomatoes, Strawberries, Watermelon

Orange: Apricot, Butternut Squash, Carrots, Mangoes, Oranges, Peaches, Pumpkin

Yellow: Bananas, Chamomile, Corn, Grapefruit, Lemons, Yellow Squash

Green: Asparagus, Avocados, Celery, Green Beans, Kale, Lettuce, Mint, Peas

Blue: Blueberries, Blue Corn
Indigo: Black Beans, Blackberry, Boysenberries, Plums, Prunes
Violet: Cabbage, Eggplant, Elderberries, Lavender, Passionfruit, Purple (Red) Onions

4. Chew your food thoroughly.

This is an often overlooked health topic, but the reasoning behind the suggestion makes a lot of sense, and chewing thoroughly definitely leads to better health.

Chewing your food thoroughly brings many benefits. First, it slows down your meal, and that alone brings two main benefits. 1. It slows the release of sugar into your system. When your sugar level spikes quickly, that will be followed by a corresponding quick insulin spike, which will lower your blood sugar. That's a guarantee of one thing: that you will soon crave a quick carb fix to get your sugar back up. That one rushed meal will begin a vicious cycle. 2. Your brain has a built in hunger-stopping mechanism. When you've eaten enough food, the brain sends a signal that it's time to stop eating. But that satiation signal has a little built-in time delay. If you eat too quickly, you'll have eaten several bites before the signal has time to take effect. That leads to overeating, which, for your health, is never a good thing.

But chewing thoroughly brings other important benefits. Your digestive system has quite a workload in digesting food. Where does the digestive system begin? In the mouth. The rest of the digestive system is literally at the mercy of the mouth, because only the mouth has a voluntary role in digestion. Once the food gets past the mouth, it's all involuntary from there. But when you make the decision to chew your food thoroughly, you are aiding the digestive process in two ways:

First, and probably foremost, chewing to break food down into small particles is absolutely vital to good digestion. Your teeth are designed to do that; your stomach is not. If you were to forego chewing, the rest of the digestive system would have its workload multiplied exponentially. And still, it could not do as thorough a job as it could if the food were well chewed. (This creates a huge energy drain on your body's resources. Would you rather spend your energy in play, in getting essential work done, in spending time with your friends and family, or would you rather spend it digesting food that you've neglected to chew?)

Second, saliva is loaded with substances that start the process of digestion right in the mouth. By breaking your food down with your teeth and saturating it with saliva, your digestive process gets a huge head start and has a much easier workload.

As an example, think, if you will, about eating a handful of cashews. Cashews are dry, solid, and have a definite shape. But when you chew them, they quickly turn into a moist smooth paste. That's very easy work for your mouth. Picture both scenarios now: either those dry, hard, whole cashews reaching your stomach, or the smooth cashew paste you've made with your mouth doing so. I'm sure you can see the difference from your stomach's point of view. What in the world will it do with those whole cashews, or even cashew pieces for that matter? It doesn't have teeth and can't do the job. That food will remain largely undigested and a burden to the system.

To further illustrate the benefits of thorough chewing, you might want to try this: Get a nice, juicy, sweet apple. Honeycrisp work well for this, especially when they are in season. Either take a bite of the apple or cut a slice and put it in your mouth. Then begin to chew the apple as you focus on the taste sensation in your mouth. Don't swallow any of the pulp; just chew on the apple pieces and pay attention to the juice being separated from the pulp.

When the juice has been completely extracted and swallowed, then you may swallow the pulp.

What will you find? If the apple is a high quality apple with good texture, taste, and sweetness, you'll notice how quickly the juice is extracted from the pulp when you chew. And that juice is sweet, delightful, and the freshest juice you'll ever taste. And when you've finished each "sip" of the juice (each mouthful), you'll chase that down with the pulp, or fiber, which brings additional health benefits. Your taste buds, your brain, your digestive system, and your entire body get a delightful treat.

But now think about what happens if you merely chew that piece of apple only a few times, just enough to break it up so the pieces are small enough to swallow. The juice is not extracted from the pulp, and those pieces end up in your stomach, in a wet, acidic environment, sitting there for hours at 98.6 degrees Fahrenheit (37 degrees Celsius) before they can be digested. Do you think you'll be getting any benefits of fresh raw juice that way?

There's an old saying: "Drink your solids and chew your liquids." That's actually excellent advice. Give your body a break by chewing your foods thoroughly. Your body will thank you . . . not verbally, of course, but with extra energy and in many other ways.

5. Keep plenty of healthful foods on hand; keep junk foods out of the home if possible.

You know the routine . . . it's mid-afternoon, you get hungry, and you decide to eat something healthful as your snack. Perhaps a nice small salad with lettuce, onions, carrots, tomatoes, and avocados, topped with a little canned tuna. You open the fridge, and the only lettuce you see is an old head of iceberg, clearly past its prime. You have one-half onion, but no carrots or tomatoes, and you have two avocados . . . one is as hard as a baseball and the other one clearly passed the guacamole stage two weeks earlier. There's no tuna in the pantry either. But while you are in the refrigerator you notice one of your favorite cupcakes. What's going to happen next? We both know the answer to that.

It's often overlooked, but a key to dietary success is to have the right foods on hand. Having them prepared in advance, if possible, is even better. We are trying to balance three factors: 1. We want to eat healthier foods and to be healthier. 2. We want our food to taste good. 3. We are busy people, and realistically, convenience is usually going to win. You can stack the odds of success in your favor by having healthful, tasty, nutritious foods in the home and as ready to eat as possible.

The same principle applies when you are away from home. Having a bag of seeds, nuts, some fruit, raw vegies, or something else you like will get you out of many jams and keep your diet on track.

6. Don't eat more than a snack late in the evening.

Your diet and your sleep are intertwined. Have a bad night's sleep, or hardly get any sleep, and for most people that's the perfect storm to eat the wrong foods and to eat too much of them the following day.

What's one of the surest ways to get a bad night's sleep? Eat a large meal late in the evening. Why is this so? The body and the brain both need and crave quality sleep, but they are only able to get quality sleep when they can truly rest. Digesting a meal is a huge task for both the body and brain. How so? The body spends much energy in digesting and processing food. Virtually all of the major organs are involved and at work; digestion is like a symphony between many organs. And the brain? It's the conductor of that symphony, and it must be alert to direct everything that's going on.

The body needs to do a few things while asleep, and that's essentially to rest, to heal, to cleanse, and to renew. The brain needs to do gazillions of things, including rest, process the days events, and dream about any myriads of things, some of which are logical and some of which defy logic. If your brain is busy with the digestion process, it won't get the rest it needs, and it won't be able to do the fun stuff you need, such as dreaming.

So by eating a meal late at night, we initiate a dangerous cycle: Poor night sleep, fatigue during the day, overeating, including late at night, another poor night's sleep, and so on. Break that cycle by, as a general practice, refraining from eating more than a snack past, perhaps, 7:00 pm.

7. Consider organic foods.

When I first heard about organic foods, I was perhaps in middle school in the late 1960s. The concept seemed odd to me. After all, what was wrong with the regular foods we'd been eating?

To my parents and especially grandparents, the concept of organic foods would have been really odd. Not too long ago foods were grown on family-run farms in mostly organic fashion. But beginning perhaps in the early-to-mid 1900s, and escalating ever since, farming techniques have relied on chemicals to make crops more pest-resistant and more profitable. Profitable, in this case, means larger, heavier, altered produce.

However, there has been a weighty price to pay for such tampering. The foods retain some of the chemicals, lose much of their nutritional value, and in other ways they are poor imitations of the original, natural foods.

Try the banana test! This point really hit home with me not too long ago with bananas. Simply put, I realized that as a child I liked bananas. They were not my favorite fruit, but they were still pretty high up there on the list. And yet, through the years, I noticed I had eaten less and less bananas until, in recent years, I stopped eating them completely. I never gave this much thought until my wife mentioned how bananas have changed: they didn't taste like they used to. She too had stopped eating bananas in the meantime, referring to them as overly large, rubbery, and chemically tasting. That was exactly how I'd describe them too.

About this time my wife bought a few organic bananas. I tried one and could not believe what I was tasting. The banana was soft, and it actually tasted like . . . a banana, which was a flavor I had almost forgotten about through the years. This proved to be no fluke, as we've been eating organic bananas since, and every one has that soft, mellow, unique banana flavor we loved so much as children. Some organic foods are worth the extra money if you can afford them. I'll never eat another bloated "rubber-chemical banana" again.

8. Don't overeat.

Eating, needless to say, is very good for our health. Overeating is very bad for our health. Sadly, many people formed an overeating habit early in life, often at the encouragement of their parents to 'clean their plate.' Instead of eating to satisfaction, they eat until they are full . . . okay, stuffed. And they do this pretty much at every meal, and even all day long. What are the results?

Go to your local Walmart or wherever else the general public gathers and look around. Obesity is an epidemic, and it's not getting better. Some people, in a mere thirty or forty years of life, are so large that they can't even walk, and if they can, it's with great difficulty. Usually when they get to that point, there's almost no turning back. (But it can be done by some who possess great motivation and moxie.)

Notice please some of the problems caused by frequent overeating:

Obesity
Heart Disease
Diabetes
High Cholesterol
High Blood Pressure
Stroke
Cancer
Excessive doctor's visits
Digestive Disorders
Social Issues and Low Self-Esteem
Lower-Body Joint Pain
Heartburn
Exhaustion
Back and Spine Problems
Knee Problems
Financial Problems, Including Frequent Wardrobe
    Adjustments
Lack of Physical Conditioning
Loss of Mobility
Mood Swings
Guilt
Preoccupation with Body Weight
Early Death

Stop the trend now. Remember, gaining only one pound per month will get you in trouble fast. That's 12 pounds a year, 48 pounds in four years, 120 pounds in ten years, and I won't even mention the numbers for thirty or forty years.

One of the best ways to avoid overeating is to eat slowly and chew well. That extends your time with a meal, providing more enjoyment with less food, and it allows the hunger stop-signal to kick in before you've downed another 350 unnecessary calories. Working with the body's signals and rhythms is to your benefit. Overeating, clearly is not.

9. If you fall off the bandwagon, get right back on.

It's the rare person who does not "cheat" on a diet. But those who are successful know how to "cheat" and then immediately get back on track. A reasonable cheat here and there won't submarine your health, but remaining in the dietary gutter will.

At times you may want to plan in advance to cheat. Suppose you are attending a wedding or some other gala event. Have a plan in advance. Know how far off your diet you are willing to go for the occasion, and then be determined to get right back on it the next day. Such planning can save lots of dietary blowouts, crashes, and heartaches.

10. Stay educated about health and nutrition.

One of the best ways to eat a healthy diet is to read about healthy diets and to read about health in general. There are two main reasons:

a. **When you read about health and healthy dieting, you are educating (and arming) yourself.** If you choose your reading material wisely, and you read with discernment, you'll be consistently learning more about the principles and logic of good nutrition. Armed with that knowledge, you can make better choices. I'm pleased to report that there is now an abundance of excellent publications that teach principles of sound health. That wasn't always the case. When choosing reading material, avoid fad-like material and focus on what are sound principles of health and nutrition, ones that are backed by logic and that work in harmony with the body's natural cycles and rhythms.

b. **Reading about health is very motivating.** It's amazing how just thirty minutes with a good health book can cause a person to change their diet, their exercise routines, and so forth. When you need a good health boost, read about healthy living. It's very motivating, and you'll likely soon be on a better path.

Of course, there is a need to be selective about what you read . . . Wonder Bread did not really build bodies 12 ways, Wheaties may be the "Breakfast of Champions," but is it really the breakfast of champions, literally? Some of the old food pyramids were absurd. My home economics teacher in high school told our class that ice cream is about the perfect food, because it contains everything important: dairy, protein, fats, carbohydrates, calcium, and often fruit. And Wiley Brooks, leader of the Breatherian movement, which claims we can get all the nutrients we need just from the air we breathe, was caught, well, you guessed it, sneaking out for a late-night binge on junk food.

So when you select your reading material, look for those sources that offer a balanced approach to nutrition. Specifically, does the diet seem to be in harmony with the way our bodies are designed? If not, it's best to look elsewhere.

Kindle books have changed the way we can shop for our reading material. You can download a sample of almost any book. Look through the sample, and if you find that the book is to your liking and can benefit you in your quest for better health, then you can buy the book on Kindle, which is usually less expensive than the paperback versions.

11. Eat living foods.

Living foods refer to foods that still have life in them, such as enzymes. These include raw (uncooked) foods, sprouted foods, and cultured foods. The enzymes in living foods help your body in several ways. Once those foods are heated to a certain degree, the enzymes are damaged and can thus provide no benefit.

Think of the difference between eating a raw food and a cooked food, such as green peppers, carrots, or apples. While those foods are delicious when they are cooked and healthful to a degree, you can tell as you're chewing them that they are not living. There's no crunch, and the subtle taste of the raw flavors are no longer there. It's the same difference between drinking raw juices or eating soup. Soup is healthful, but if you really want to treat your body to a health boost, there's nothing like raw juice. It's alive, and it will give your body more life, more spark.

Some foods are better cooked, some even need to be cooked. For instance, I'm not about to dine on uncooked pinto beans or artichokes. And while I have eaten raw potatoes, there's no question that I prefer them cooked. (And my guess is that at least 99% of those who read that statement feel the same way.) Don't be fanatical about living foods, feeling that you are breaking a law by eating cooked foods. Just be sure to eat a good amount of living foods in your daily diet. It makes a difference.

12. Don't skip breakfast, and make it a high-protein meal.

One of the best recent trends among nutritionists is to recommend that we eat high-protein breakfasts. It makes a lot of sense. Breakfasts have increasingly become a carbohydrate-fest. Throw that quick energy down the gullet and buzz out the door. It feels pretty good at the time, but in about an hour or two you have stopped buzzing and it doesn't feel so good anymore. The stage is actually set for a day of dietary misery and weight gain.

Dietary misery and weight gain? Yes. A high-carbohydrate breakfast, such as dry cereal with milk and sugar, a Danish, and a glass of orange juice, will provide an immediate spike in blood sugar. Such a meal has a drug-like effect on the body, as the quick high is followed by a quick low. And there's only one way to fix that quick low . . . get another quick high. How? Another high-carb meal. If you eat a high-carb breakfast, the roller coaster effect of high and low sugar will begin for the day. That's exhausting to the body, and it packs on the pounds.

A high-protein breakfast sets the stage for a day of balanced meals. Protein doesn't provide the spike in sugar that carbohydrates do—the protein meal sustains you much longer—so you'll be much less prone to cravings for sweets during the day.

A high-protein breakfast does not mean an ALL-protein breakfast. It's good to include a small-to-moderate amount of carbohydrates and fat. So what constitutes a good breakfast? Aim for at least 20-25 grams of protein, and limit the fat content to perhaps 10-15 grams and the carbohydrate amount to 15-25 grams, or perhaps higher if you are very physically active. So a breakfast of 2-3 eggs or a few ounces of animal protein, a small serving of cooked cereal, with a little olive oil on the cereal, and a small piece of fruit (perhaps a few slices of an apple, a few slices of a banana, or some berries) may be about ideal.

Keep in mind that you don't have to have your breakfast the moment you get out of bed. But if you need a quick pickup, you can start your day with perhaps a handful of nuts or seeds or a small piece of fruit. Then, perhaps thirty to sixty minutes later, you can have your full breakfast. Listen to your body and see what works best for you.

Some people simply don't have much of an appetite in the morning, and others don't have the time or inclination to prepare a meal when they first wake up. A good solution: One of my favorite nutritionists recommends a protein drink for breakfast. I often do this. I'll use a base of perhaps unsweetened coconut milk, add in about 25 grams of a good protein powder, add a helping of sunflower seeds, then perhaps a teaspoon of honey, and finally some non-glycemic sweetener, such as a combination of monk fruit and erythritol. You can also add some fruit to your shake. The morning protein shake is quick, it's nutritious, it's tasty, and it's a great dietary start to the day.

13. Consider eating probiotics.

This is one topic that is gaining increasing attention in recent years. And for good reason. So much of our well-being is determined by what is known as our "gut health." So what are probiotics, and how do they help us?

Probiotics are healthy bacteria. (*Pro* means "for" and *biota* means "life".) We need these bacteria in abundance in our digestive systems. There are an estimated (have fun trying to do an exact count!) 100 trillion microorganisms, from 500 unique species, in the normal healthy human bowel. Most of these are healthful, and they keep harmful microorganisms, known as "pathogens," from taking over and damaging our bodies.

Probiotics do a world of wonder for us: They not only fight pathogens, but they aid in digestion, nutrient absorption, and they boost immune function. In other words, you've got trillions of tiny friendly helpers working to make your life easier and your health better. Without these helpers you are more prone to several ailments of the digestive system, such as constipation, diarrhea, and urinary tract infections (UTIs), as well as other ailments, such as skin disorders.

Modern living and modern diet can severely reduce the amount of probiotics in the intestinal system. How can you boost your probiotic count? There are two basic ways:

a. Eat fermented foods that boost your probiotics.

The best sources of probiotic foods are foods that have been fermented. Fermented dairy products include yogurt, kefir, and buttermilk. Other fermented foods high in probiotics are non-dairy yogurts, such as those made from soy and coconut milk, sourdough bread, kimchi, sauerkraut and other pickled vegetables, and kombucha. Currently, several of our close friends are making their own kombucha, and they enjoy the process thoroughly.

b. Take probiotic supplements.

Taking probiotic supplements can also add to the count of friendly bacteria in your body. Look for probiotics that are sold refrigerated, and continue to refrigerate your probiotics when you bring them home. Notice that the count of supplemental probiotics is often over 25 billion per capsule.

14. If you have food allergies, avoid the foods you are allergic to.

Have you heard about food allergies? Are you skeptical? There's no need to be. Food allergies are real, and they can wreak havoc on our bodies (and minds).

Some food allergies are very obvious. For instance, a small group of people are allergic to peanuts, and the allergy is severe. Just one peanut, or even a pinhead size of peanut butter, can cause shock or even death. There was a news article a few years ago about a person who was allergic to shellfish, who was dining in a restaurant, when a food server merely walked by his table with a plate of steaming shellfish. Inhaling the steam alone caused that person to die.

Most food allergies are less severe and less noticeable, and they create less of a problem, but they can still do a number on us, especially over time. Common allergens are wheat, dairy, eggs, peanuts, shellfish, and many others.

How do you know if you have a food allergy? There are many methods of testing for food allergies. But even without testing, there are often very clear signs that would indicate an allergy to a certain food. One sign is very obvious: You likely are allergic to a food if, after eating it, you consistently develop a specific physical symptom. So if you break out in a rash every time you eat, say, products with corn, you are almost surely allergic to corn. My easiest allergy to detect is aged cheese. If I eat some parmesan, feta, or other aged cheese, my skin will begin to itch almost immediately. Then when I wake up the next day, my IQ seems to drop in half, as my brain feels like it's wrapped in a thick fog. It's no fun, and I avoid aged cheese at virtually all costs. (I desperately miss those 30 IQ points when that happens.)

But there is another sign of being allergic to a food that is a little trickier—actually, it's a lot trickier: If there is a food that you are repeatedly drawn back to, because you love eating it and it immediately makes you feel better, such as more energized, you likely are allergic to that food. Keep in mind that we all have food preferences. We simply like certain foods more than others, and that's natural. But if our pull to a certain food is unusually strong, to where that food is almost a must for us each day and perhaps each meal, we may be allergic to it. But why is that so? Why would we be drawn to a food we are allergic to?

As with sugar addiction, it all gets back to adrenal hits. When we eat the offending food, our body reacts to it. But the reaction to this food is not so noticeable and it actually feels good, not bad. No rash, no headache, no itching, etc. Our body reacts by trying to neutralize the damage from the food, so it releases extra cortisol and adrenaline. That provides a "rush" to our system, and it seems to give us more energy, which feels good. But as with a sugar "rush," in a short while we are weaker than we were before the rush. How can we feel better again? Only one way: eat more of that same food for another rush. And the cycle has begun: Eat the offending food, get an energy rush, come down from that rush to a lower level, eat the offending food again, another rush, and so on.

If you remember my aged cheese allergy: I have no desire to eat aged cheese at all. But I also have a strong chocolate allergy. Do I have a desire to eat chocolate? There are three answers to that question: Yes, YES, and, **YES**. Okay, there is a fourth answer: **YES!** If I could, I'd eat chocolate all day every day. Semi-dark 50% cocoa will do just fine, thank you. In fact, once I begin eating chocolate, it's extremely difficult to stop. And I want my next meal to be . . . more chocolate, not to mention several chocolate snacks in between. My allegery/addiction is so strong that I have decided to forego eating chocolate at all. Just one bite and my health suffers from the inevitable roller coaster addiction again.

If you learn what foods you're allergic to, and you avoid them, your body will be spared from the constant ups and downs of the adrenal hits caused by those foods and eventual adrenal exhaustion. If you don't avoid them completely, please know that the more you do avoid them, the less stress there will be on your body.

True Story: You may have caught it, or you may not have, but I placed the fourth "**YES!**", the large one, in a dark brown font to replicate the color of chocolate. (This will be evident in Kindle editions of this book but not paperback copies, which are printed in black and white.) Just to show you how strong a food allergy/addiction can be, a day or so after changing the color of the font, when I went back to add to this section, I noticed that font, and I actually began to instantly crave dark chocolate—just from the color alone. The point: food allergies are real, and if you crave a certain food inordinately, you likely are allergic to it. Even though it makes you feel better when you first eat it, that allergy could be undermining your health and well-being. It may be good to be checked for food allergies if you have this dilemma.

15. Drink plenty of water.

It's been said millions of times before, and it's worth repeating . . . make sure to drink enough high-quality water on a daily basis to meet your body's needs. The human body needs to stay well-hydrated to function at its best. How much water is enough? Of course, it depends on several factors, such as your body weight, your level of activity, the climate you live in, and so on. But there are some good rules of thumb that will work, especially as a minimum, for most people.

One of these rules is to drink at least half of your body weight in ounces on a daily basis. So if you weigh 200 pounds, you should drink at least 100 ounces of water per day.

If you are like me and many others, you may find that it's difficult to drink that much water, especially out of a glass or cup. The solution? Drinking out of a water bottle, especially where you use a spout, or where your entire mouth can cover the drinking area, such as a common water bottle, makes it much easier, and more enjoyable, to drink our daily water needs.

As a suggestion, it's best to drink the vast amount of your daily water during the day. Drinking too much water at night, and especially close to bedtime, will have a detrimental effect on your sleep. Running to the bathroom several times a night, and constantly interrupting and restarting your sleep cycles, is not restful.

Finally, listen to and obey your thirst. It's been said that when you feel thirsty, you have already been clinically dehydrated for some time. I may not be the most interesting man in the world, but I can offer this: Don't stay thirsty, my friends. That thirst signal is there for a reason . . . quench it.

16. Be Peaceful, Forgiving, Thankful, Generous, and Loving.

What do being peaceful, forgiving, thankful, generous, and loving have to do with diet and health? A lot, because they are all intertwined with your health and ultimately your diet too. Let's take a look at these five qualities as they relate to health.

Peaceful. If we are peaceful in our relationships with others, our minds will be calmer and more at peace. And when our minds are calmer and more at peace, so are our hearts, nerves, and stomachs. Meals will be more pleasant, you'll probably eat more slowly, and your food will be digested much better. Thus, you'll reap more benefits from your diet.

While it's good to be peaceful, it's even more beneficial to be a peace seeker. Look for ways to resolve situations that may arise, perhaps even choosing to let things go that are not really serious. Some like to fight every little thing because, they say, it's the principle involved. But there's also the principle that humans should live peaceful, happy, and healthy lives. Not making issues of smaller things is a good way to accomplish that.

Forgiving. Hanging on to resentment is, simply put, awful for your health. It's been wisely said that holding resentment inside is the equivalent of drinking poison and then waiting for the other person to die. When you hold on to resentment, you <u>may</u> or <u>may not</u> injure the other person, but you <u>always</u> injure yourself. The major damage is always to you. Resentment will have a negative effect on your stress levels, your disposition, your relationships with family and friends, your blood pressure levels, your pulse rate, your sleep, probably your diet, and many other important aspects of life.

It's been said that "marriage is the union of two good forgivers." That same principle applies to all friendships. If you are reasonable and forgiving, you'll have more friends, and that in itself is a huge stress reliever that will benefit your health.

Thankful. A classic example of one who is not thankful is a spoiled child who thinks that the world owes him anything he wants and that everything revolves around him. The child is thankful for nothing (because, remember, it's owed to him), and he is definitely of ill temper and manner and may even throw tantrums when he doesn't get his way. You may have noticed that spoiled children are never happy children.

And this brings us to adults. Some of us never fully grow out of the childish mold just mentioned. We may not literally jump up and down and throw things when we don't get our way, but we find other creative ways to pout and make ourselves miserable.

Learning to be thankful for what we have, and maintaining reasonable expectations of others, is a great way to keep our peace and to take greater pleasure in what we have, including our food and meals. That leads, of course, to better health physically, mentally, and emotionally.

Generous. Being generous is a wonderful way to live. The generous person cares about others and looks for ways to help them or to lighten their load. Such a giving spirit is usually returned to us by others. (But please don't fall into the trap of believing that everyone we show generosity to will be properly appreciative of our kind acts. In today's world, sadly, that's not going to happen.) Many health experts recommend generosity as a way to increase your own personal happiness, not to mention the positive effect on the recipients of our kindness.

And remember, there are many ways to be generous. One obvious way is with material resources and gifts. But there are other ways of displaying generosity: giving of our time, our energy, our affection, even just our warm smiles—these are all forms of generosity that pay dividends. If we are generous, we'll not only sleep better, we'll also eat (and assimilate what we eat) better. That means better health and more energy.

Loving. Love is the pinnacle of good qualities. Work hard to develop a loving disposition. This includes kind acts, but it also includes how we view others. Do we tend to focus on their weaknesses and mistakes, or do we focus on their good qualities? Are we patient, or are we quick to take offense? The loving person looks for the best in every person and every situation. They then try to achieve the best outcome possible.

And don't neglect to be loving to yourself. It would be unloving to expect more of yourself then you are capable of doing. At the same time, don't set your standards so low that you lack satisfaction in your accomplishments.

And please, never beat yourself up mentally and emotionally. It's exhausting and injurious. It's actually doubly exhausting and doubly injurious. How so?

If you think about it, when someone gets beaten up, it's exhausting to them, and they are often injured. And the person doing the beating gets exhausted and is sometimes injured as well. So if a person beats themselves up, they are assuming both roles, that of the beater and that of the beaten. That's often double the pain, double the injury, and double the exhaustion. Learn to be understanding and kind to yourself, but at the same time reasonable, with reasonable expectations. Having this point of view will pay great dividends to your health.

Yes, our personal qualities make a difference to our health.

17. Consider these excellent diets.

In this chapter, I have offered many tips that lead to better dietary practices. While you can probably form a diet based on the information in this chapter, I haven't really outlined a specific diet. I don't believe that's my place, and I have zero desire to add a bunch of recipes to this book. It's just not what I do, which is write mostly about logic: the logic of how to play Sudoku, the logic of how to be an effective writer, the logic of eating a healthy, balanced diet, and so forth. And besides, there are many superb nutrition books on the market that teach specific diets.

Three of my very favorites are The Adrenal Reset Diet, The Mediterranean Diet, and The Schwarzbein Principle. Why do I favor these diets? They all "get it": They are among the most balanced in their approach to diet, they are founded by experts, and they are in harmony with the unbreakable relationship between natural food and the human body. These diets all completely ignore and run counter to the typical American diet, and the results are something that is not a usual outcome of the typical American diet: **robust health.**

Are these three diets drastically different from each other? Not at all. In fact, they are very similar to each other. Why? Because they are all based on sound principles of good nutrition; therefore, they all have many common threads running through them. Adhering to any of these three diets is almost guaranteed to bring you better health. Let's take a quick look at all three diets:

Adrenal Reset Diet

The Adrenal Reset Diet, created by Dr. Alan Christianson, may be my favorite of all the published diets. Alan Christianson is a genius in the field of nutrition, and his book, *The Adrenal Reset Diet*, is a *New York Times* bestseller.

What are the highlights of the diet? First, of course, all foods eaten should be natural and healthful. But the crux of the diet is perhaps the concept of carbohydrate cycling. This refers to the practice of starting the day with a high-protein, low-carbohydrate meal, and then increasing carbohydrate intake as the day progresses. (Dr. Christianson points out that it's not only *what* you eat that is important, but also *when* you eat it.)

This way of eating works in harmony with the body's natural cycles, as carbs are not as necessary early in the day when the cortisol levels are at their peak, but they become more important as the day goes on and the cortisol levels slope downward. Further, eating too many carbohydrates early in the day starts the process of blood sugar highs and resulting lows for the entire day. A higher protein breakfast gets your day off to a smoother start, and it prevents those sugar spikes and the ensuing carbohydrate cravings.

Dr. Christianson, on the bio on his excellent web site, says: "I learned that my gift was being able to quickly digest huge amounts of information, comparing it against my experience, and synthesising new perspectives out of it." He is not exaggerating. His approach to nutrition and health is about as natural, well thought out, reasonable, and brilliant as I've ever seen.

Dr. Christianson has set up wonderful web programs for those seeking better health, and he strongly believes in health education. If you sign up for his web program, you'll be treated to a wealth of superb information. Dr. Christianson also has a strong video presence on the web. He is a teacher of health and nutrition issues extraordinaire.

As much as I love the Adrenal Reset Diet, I'm also excited about Dr. Christianson's new book, *The Metabolism Reset Diet*, due to be released on January 29, 2019. This is one nature-oriented doctor who totally gets it, and I highly recommend him and his work.

The Mediterranean Diet

The *U.S. News and World Report* assembled a team of experts to study and rank the top 40 best-known diets. In the categories of Best Diet for Healthy Eating and Best Diet Overall, guess which one came in last? Yep, the keto diet. But which one was crowned the healthiest diet? Actually, it was a two-way tie between the D.A.S.H diet and the Mediterranean diet. I give the nod to the Mediterranean diet. It's easier to follow and feels more natural. It also feels less "medical" and more romantic. The diet is based on the lifestyles of the healthiest people of the Mediterranean region. This includes parts of such countries as Italy, France, Spain, Greece, Morocco, and Portugal. The key features of the diet are to eat natural, unprocessed foods as often as possible. Such foods as vegetables, fruits, olive oil, beans, nuts, seeds, grains, herbs, and spices form the bulk of the diet. Fish and seafood should be eaten often, at least two times a week. Moderate portions of poultry, eggs, cheese, and yogurt can be eaten daily or weekly. Meats, such as beef and pork, should be eaten less often, or sparingly. Sweets should also be eaten sparingly.

Finally, the Mediterranean diet stresses such non-dietary issues as spending time with friends, eating meals together, relaxing together, and engaging in healthful physical activity.

It's clear from the above description that the Mediterranean diet is natural and healthy. There is an abundance of good books on the market that explain the diet in detail.

You may find the Mediterranean Diet Pyramid, below, helpful. You can order a poster of the pyramid, download a free PDF, or even order a magnet to stick on your refrigerator. Thus, every time you open that door you'll be reminded of the importance of eating in this healthful and enjoyable way. For posters, PDFs, and magnets, contact Oldways, a non-profit organization that is dedicated to teaching people how to eat a healthier, more natural diet, at www.oldwayspt.org/medpyramid.

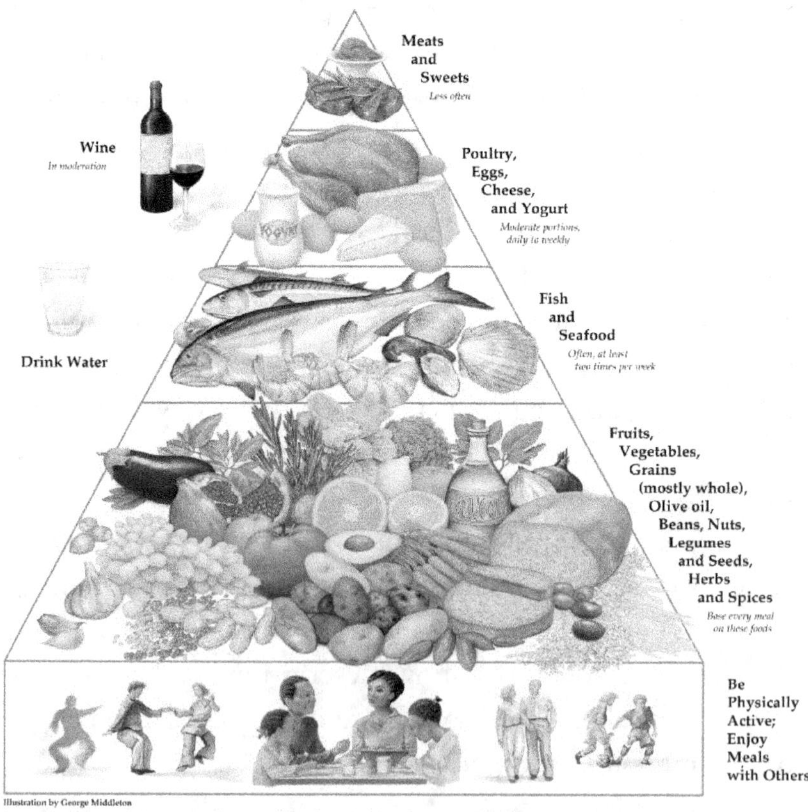

The Schwarzbein Principle

The Schwarzbein Principle is the lesser-known of the three diets I've chosen to highlight. It's just never really gotten as much of the public eye as the others. There may be a few reasons.

One, Diana Schwarzbein, founder of the Schwarzbein Principle, is a renowned endocrinologist, and her books, such as *The Schwarzbein Principle* and *The Schwarzbein Principle II*, are much more than just diet books. They are actually medical journals that expertly explain the relationship between diet and the endocrine glands and their hormones. Dr. Schwarzbein provides a remarkably thorough explanation of how insulin, thyroid, and cortisol all function, and she teaches how to improve their effectiveness.

Two, there is an abundance of books, by an abundance of authors, that explain the Adrenal Reset Diet and the Mediterranean diet. Because the Schwarzbein Principle is clearly the property of Dr. Schwarzbein, other authors have not piggybacked on the diet by publishing recipe books and further explanations of the diet. In that way, it's kept a lower profile.

Finally, the word "diet" is not included in the title of *The Schwarzbein Principle*. Those searching for diet books will be less likely to find Dr. Schwarzbein's books.

Nevertheless, Dr. Schwarzbein is a brilliant doctor, nutritionist, and writer. Her understanding of the principles of a healthy diet are spot on, and she explains why, very clearly, fad diets such as the keto diet are dangerous.

Dr. Christianson and Dr. Schwarzbein have something in common that is important to note. Both struggled with severely poor health in their youth. It was that struggle that caused them to put so much of their energy into learning the ins and outs of the effects of diet on human health. And their passion for their work is clearly fueled by their own personal experiences.

But If You Insist On Doing Keto, Consider These Suggestions

If it were my choice, I'd suggest that, unless your physician has instructed otherwise, you leave the keto diet and begin one of the healthier diets. That said, if you do stay on keto, you can make adjustments to ensure that your keto diet is as healthy as possible. Here are the steps:

1. Focus on micronutrients as well as macronutrients.

In other words, pay close attention to not only the amounts of proteins, fats, and carbohydrates that you eat, but also pay close attention to ensure that you are eating a variety of healthful foods that contain lots of vitamins, minerals, enzymes, and the like. Eat the rainbow. And remember, you can eat a virtually unlimited amount of most raw vegetables on the keto diet. Don't neglect that provision.

2. Eat healthy fats.

There's a lot of published information on what constitutes healthy fats. There's even a book entitled "Good Fat, Bad Fat." Essentially, fats from vegetable sources are considered healthy, and saturated fats from animal sources are considered not healthy. Especially favor good fats, such as olive oil, and definitely avoid harmful trans fats. (Trans fats are found in many processed foods.)

3. Eat as many carbohydrates as your keto diet allows.

Many versions of the keto diet allow up to fifty grams of carbohydrate consumption daily. Remember, carbs are not the enemy. It's not a case of the less you eat . . . you win. So do eat and enjoy every one of those fifty grams. Fifty grams of carbs a day is still lacking to be completely healthy for the long term, but it's much healthier than, say, twenty or thirty grams per day, which is a severe restriction of a nutrient your body needs.

4. Carb up at night.

Does it matter when you eat most of your carbohydrates? Apparently so, according to many nutritionists, including some who advocate the keto diet. The experts suggest beginning the day with a relatively low-carb breakfast (but not "no-carb"), then increasing the amounts of carbohydrates for the noon meal, and then finally eating an even more generous supply of carbohydrates with their supper. Why?

When you first wake in the morning, your cortisol levels are normally at their highest point of the day. As your cortisol levels drop throughout the day, there is a greater need for carbohydrates to supply energy.

Further, by beginning your day with a high-carbohydrate meal, a cycle begins. Your blood sugar will quickly rise, and then insulin will cause it to quickly drop, then you'll need to quickly raise it again, then it will drop, and so on. So let's say that your goal is fifty grams of carbohydrates per day, and let's say that you are eating three meals per day. At breakfast you may want to have 10 grams of carbohydrates, at the noon meal you may want to eat 15 grams of carbohydrates, and at supper time you may want to eat 25 grams of carbohydrates. This pattern of increasing carbohydrate consumption as the day progresses is known as "carb cycling."

5. Follow the healthful eating guidelines, to the degree possible, as outlined in the chapter "A Better Approach to Diet."

The chapter "A Better Approach to Diet" is loaded with tips that will help you to eat a healthier diet and to eat in a more health-building way. I suggest you follow the principles in that chapter as closely as possible.

Are Keto Authors and Advocates Trying to Pull One Over on You?

No, they're not. Not at all. They are sincere in their efforts to help you. Put yourself in their situation.

For instance, one keto author, a woman, consumed enormous amounts of soda and other carbohydrates every day and all day, and she weighed 289 pounds when she began the keto diet. She lost slightly over 100 pounds in her first year on the diet, and then she continued to drop additional weight until she was a healthful 168 pounds. For a woman of her height—five feet, eleven inches—that's excellent. And her book features many before and after photos—the difference is stunning. I showed one of the "after" pictures to my wife, and with great emphasis she said exactly what I was thinking: "She's beautiful." Truly, she looks like a completely different person, and she reports that her life has been greatly benefitted.

If that were you, what would you do? Probably, if you liked to write, you'd hit the word processor and hit it with zeal. And that's exactly the case with so many keto book writers. They are thrilled at the transformation in their lives, and they want to let you enjoy the same benefits they're reaping. That's very kind of them and commendable.

For these authors, the keto diet may have been a life-saver. But as I've shown throughout this book, the keto diet is deficient and full of potential dangers, especially long-term dangers. These authors have experienced how the keto diet has helped them, but they are unaware of those long-term dangers. There are better, safer, more natural ways to lose weight and to achieve and maintain vibrant health than the keto diet.

Note: Why do these people seem to thrive on the keto diet? It's because they have actually upgraded their diet. Upgraded their diet? But wasn't the keto diet rated as the least healthy diet among the forty diets ranked by *The U.S. News and World Report*?

Yes, it was. But there was one diet that was not included in the rankings that is worse than the keto diet. Which diet is that? The "junk food diet" that is so typical in the Western World. If I had to make a personal choice between spending some time on the keto diet or a diet that is laden with deep fried foods, trans fat, and loaded with sugar, I'd select the keto diet.

Furthermore, because they were "on a diet" and were trying to lose weight, they were likely much more careful to control their portions and intake than those who are just eating whatever they want whenever they want it.

Research, Quotes, and Thoughts

The U.S. News and World Report assembled a team of experts who conducted a comprehensive study and comparison of forty of the most popular diets in 2018. The study ranked diets according to several categories, including Best Weight Loss Diets, Best Diabetes Diets, Best Diets for Healthful Eating, Best Heart-Healthy Diets, and so forth. How did the keto diet fare?

Not so well. In fact, not good at all. Okay . . . really bad. Notice the keto diet's rankings, 1 being the best, 40 being the worst, of the forty diets:

> Best Diabetes Diet: 33rd (tie)
> Best Heart-Healthy Diet: 35th
> Best Weight-Loss Diet: 23rd
> Best Diet Overall: 39th (tie—that means it was tied for last)
> Best Diet for Healthy Eating: 40th (last)

With those ratings, maybe it's time to rethink bacon, butter, sour cream, and lard, in unlimited amounts as health foods.

Selected Quotes

"Our data suggests that animal-based low-carbohydrate diets, which are prevalent in North America and Europe, might be associated with shorter overall life span and should be discouraged," – **Sara Seidelmann, cardiologist and nutrition researcher at Brigham and Women's Hospital, Boston, Massachusetts**

"The key problem with a keto diet is it produces acid in the body . . . What's sort of scary is that [the keto diet] is an experiment that the population is doing on itself. No drug company would get away with introducing a drug in the population without thorough research." – **Edward Weiss, Kinesiologist, St. Louis University**

"To maintain your brain, muscle, bone, nerves, skin, blood circulation, and immune system, your body requires a steady supply of many different raw materials—both macronutrients and micronutrients. You need large amounts of macronutrients—proteins, fats, and carbohydrates. And while you only need a small number of micronutrients—vitamins and minerals—failing to get even those small quantities virtually guarantees disease." – *Harvard Health Publishing*, **Harvard Medical School, September 2016**

"Our study suggests that in the long-term [low-carb diets] are linked with an increased risk of death from any cause, and deaths due to cardiovascular disease, cerebrovascular disease, and cancer," – **Maciej Banach, professor at the Medical University of Lodz in Poland**

"Advocates of this type of diet [keto] give the impression that high-urine ketones are desirable and indicate success. This is not true. Furthermore, the diet is extremely dangerous because your body is breaking down tissues and causing imbalances within your system." – **Diana Schwarzbein,** *The Schwarzbein Principle*

"People on low-carb diets often turn to more butter and meat for sustenance, which can increase blood pressure and, in the case of processed meats, contribute to cancer. Meat and dairy can also contribute to inflammation in the body, which can help cancerous tumors form and grow."– **Sara Seidelmann, cardiologist and nutrition researcher at Brigham and Women's Hospital, Boston, Massachusetts**

"Banning entire food groups and thinking you can cheat your way into good health may work for a while, but it could also send you into an early grave." – **Hilary Brueck, Science Reporter** at ***Business Insider***

"The researchers also analyzed data from more than 432,000 people in more than 20 countries and found that those with high and low carbohydrate intake had shorter life expectancy than those with moderate carbohydrate intake." – **Robert Preidt, *HealthDay Reporter***

"In study after study, diet survey data from around the world reveals that people who stick to limited amounts of meats, dairy, and processed foods — and fuel up on fiber-rich plant-based foods, including vegetables, whole grains, nuts, and yes, even carb-heavy beans — have some of the best health outcomes." – **Hilary Brueck, Science Reporter at *Business Insider***

"A low-carb or high-carb diet raises your risk of death, a new study suggests, with people eating the food staple in moderation seeing the greatest benefits to their health.

"Although previous studies have shown such diets can be beneficial for short-term weight loss and lower heart risk, the longer-term impact is proving to have more negative consequences, according to the study." – **Meera Senthilingam, Global Health Journalist and London-based Editor for the CNN Health and Wellness unit.**

"Fill your plate with plants. Include vegetables, whole grains, healthy fats, and legumes. Don't include a lot of meat, milk, or highly processed foods that a gardener or farmer wouldn't recognize." – **Hilary Brueck, Science Reporter at *Business Insider***

"Three huge new studies of more than half a million people are casting major doubts on the keto diet" – **Headline, *SF Gate*, September 20, 2018**

"There's absolutely nothing more important for our health than what we eat each and every day," – **Sara Seidelmann, cardiologist and nutrition researcher at Brigham and Women's Hospital, Boston, Massachusetts**

"Should you try the keto diet? It's advertised as a weight-loss wonder, but this eating plan is actually a medical diet that comes with serious risks." –*Harvard Health Publishing*, Harvard Medical School, Harvard Health Letter, October, 2018

Summary with a Story

The keto diet reminds me of an afternoon from my high school days when I was on the track team. At a multi-school event, our team was running in the mile relay. That meant that four runners each had to cover a quarter of a mile, or one lap around the track.

One runner on our team, I'll call him Bob, was our fastest sprinter. He started his race at a very fast pace. He was way out in front, leading the rest of the runners by a large margin. That was fine, but he continued at the same pace, clearly accessing every ounce of his strength with each stride.

Those who did not know Bob may have thought they were in for a treat, for surely Bob was about to record a blistering time. But we who knew Bob were asking ourselves, "What is he doing?"

About halfway through the race you could see that Bob was slowing down. He was still running his hardest, but now the other runners were beginning to catch him. At about the 330 yard mark Bob was really struggling. He looked like he was running through a combination of drying cement, glue, and quicksand. He was still straining to run fast, but he wasn't really getting anywhere. All of the runners passed him as though he was standing still, and he was practically at walking speed (but still in running form) by the time he finished the race. It was both comical and sad.

What happened? Bob was not equipped to run the race in that manner, and probably no runner is. While it is important to get a quick start in the 440 yard run (now 400 meters), runners must relax after about six seconds, which is when they hit top speed, so as to conserve energy for the long haul. Their momentum keeps them going fast, but they are not straining and wasting energy, so that they'll have "kick" left for the latter part of the race.

We on the team also knew something about Bob that the other spectators didn't know. As fast as he was, Bob totally lacked conditioning. He not only smoked cigarettes, but he rarely trained. That didn't make a huge difference for the shorter sprints, but this was the first time Bob ran a longer distance. He was clearly not equipped for the task.

And this brings us to the keto diet. Regarding weight loss, those beginning the keto diet get a quick start. Because of mostly losing water weight from the glycogen in their muscles, the results can be stunningly fast and very encouraging. But after the initial burst, reality sets in.

The keto diet is not equipped to help them in the long run. It's lacking in essential micronutrients, it's filled with too much fat, and it's too restrictive of carbohydrates, which will leave the body under-fueled, thereby straining and running down the all-important battery system: the adrenal glands.

I think of all of those runners who passed Bob, surely enjoying every moment of doing so. They applied sound principles of running, and they were equipped for the long haul. Those who adhere to sound dietary principles, and those who follow such outstanding diets as the Adrenal Reset Diet, the Mediterranean Diet, and the Schwarzbein Principle, not only get that immediate boost when they begin the diet, but they are on a diet that is designed to balance their systems and benefit them for the long haul, their entire life. That's a winning formula. That's smart eating!

The Best of Health to You!

Other Books by David Klein

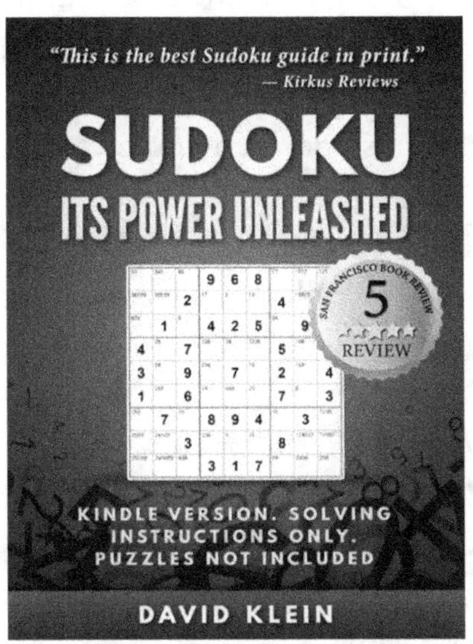

Sudoku: It's Power Unleashed, is the first of what I hope to be many Sudoku books. *Named "the best Sudoku guide in print" by Kirkus Reviews in January 2017*, the strength of this book is indeed the instruction. Learn to use many Sudoku solving methods, from the simple Only Candidate and Naked Twins, to the complex X-Wings, Y-Wings, Swordfish, and Unique Rectangles.

Five levels of puzzles are included, and candidates are provided with the puzzles, so that you can play using the most advanced methods and get to the fun and challenge of Sudoku right away.

Alphabet and Alphabet Hybrid puzzles are also a prominent feature of the book. Alphabet puzzles use letters instead of numbers, and several cells are shaded gray. When the puzzle is completed, the gray cells will spell something familiar, such as a location, book title, movie, person, food, and so on.

Alphabet Hybrid puzzles are played with numbers just like regular Sudoku puzzles, but a small conversion chart is provided where the numbers convert to letters. With a simple conversion of the shaded cells, the letters spell a location, book title, movie, person, food, and so on.

Additional hybrid puzzles include word guess, word scramble, brain playground, and math. For math puzzles, a mathematical equation is provided, with spaces for the numbers. Transfer the numbers from the shaded cells to the blanks and then complete the mathematical equation.

Note that the Kindle version of *Sudoku: Its Power Unleashed*, includes instruction only and does not include puzzles. It's not possible to play puzzles on a Kindle, which is strictly an electronic reader.

You can read the full review of *Sudoku: It's Power Unleashed*, by Kirkus Reviews. (They loved the book, awarding it a rare Kirkus star.) www.kirkusreviews.com/book-reviews/david-klein2/sudoku/

Furthermore, San Francisco Book Review awarded *Sudoku: It's Power Unleashed*, their highest rating of 5 stars.

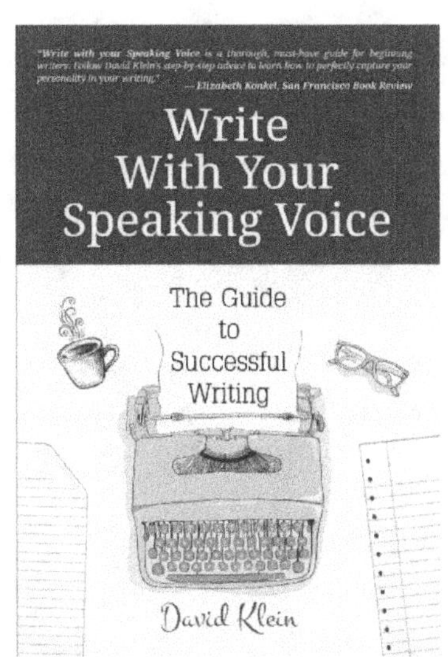

Write With Your Speaking Voice, is a writing guide for all who want to learn to write in a natural manner that matches their speaking voice. Flow-writing is explained, which allows the pattern of natural speech that flows from a speaker's mouth to instead flow to the keyboard or pen. Same speaker's patterns; same speaker's rhythms. Using your natural voice makes your writing effective; it will sound like your unique voice; it will sound like you.

Chapter titles include: Becoming a Skilled Writer, Capture Your Style of Speech, Flow-writing, Music—The Rhythm of Your Writing, Your Writing Voice, What to Write, When to Write, Writer's Block—Or Not Writer's Block, Humor, Personality, "Rules" to Put to Rest, Read Your Work Aloud, Tricky Word Choices, Self-Publishing, The Quote Collection, and many others.

Elizabeth Konkel, of the San Francisco Book Review, wrote: "*Write with your Speaking Voice* is a thorough, must-have guide for beginning writers. Follow David Klein's step-by-step advice to learn how to perfectly capture your personality in your writing."

San Francisco Book Review awarded *Write With Your Speaking Voice* their highest rating of 5 stars.

Write With Your Speaking Voice is available in Kindle and print editions.

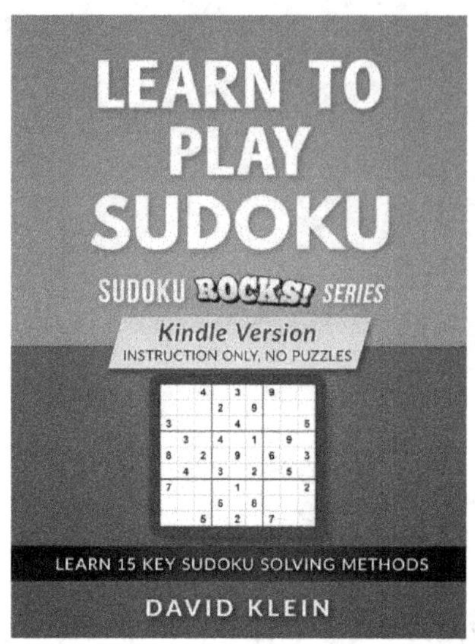

Learn to Play Sudoku rocks. It's loaded with puzzles, more than 500 of them, and they are rated at eight different levels of difficulty, including ridiculously easy to mind-boggling difficult—which are among the hardest puzzles in the world. With more than 40 pages of instruction, you'll learn to solve Sudoku puzzles more efficiently, and thus you'll enjoy playing Sudoku more and will be able to solve higher-level puzzles. (Puzzles are included in the print version only. Kindle books do not have puzzles because you can't play Sudoku on a Kindle, which is merely an electronic reader.)